Clean and Clever Doctor Jokes for Medical Professionals

BY

Aaron Remus

It is creative nonfiction, in this case. For various reasons, several parts have undergone variable degrees of fictionalization.

Copyright © Aaron Remus, 2023

Introduction

The Doctor Jokes book is a hilarious collection of humor that will tickle your funny bone and leave you in stitches. With a vibrant cover that features a cartoon doctor and stethoscope, this book is sure to catch your attention and keep you entertained. Inside, you'll find a plethora of jokes and stories that revolve around the world of medicine and healthcare. From funny one-liners about doctors and nurses to amusing anecdotes about patients and their ailments, this book is filled with laughter-inducing content. With its light-hearted tone and relatable content, the Doctor Jokes book is perfect for anyone who wants to take a break from the stresses of the medical world and have a good laugh. So whether you're a doctor, nurse, healthcare worker, or just someone who loves a good joke, this book is sure to bring a smile to your face. So go ahead and pick up a copy of the Doctor Jokes book today and get ready to laugh your way through the world of medicine!

Jokes

1. Why did the doctor carry a red pen? In case they needed to draw blood.

2. Why did the doctor always bring a rubber chicken to surgery? To use as a sterilized field.

3. Why did the doctor refuse to operate on a grape? It was already raisin' concern.

4. Why did the doctor get into the beekeeping business? They wanted to be an MD-Bee.

5. Why did the doctor give up being a chef? They didn't have the thyme.

6. Why did the doctor switch from medicine to law? They wanted to sue-cide prevention.

7. What do you call a doctor who can only perform surgery on fruit? A banana-na-na-na-na-na-na-na-na-na-na-na-na-na-na-na-na Doctor!

8. Why did the doctor become an archaeologist? They wanted to keep digging up old problems.

9. Why did the doctor refuse to see the pirate? They didn't take insurance that had a high co-pay.

10. What did the doctor say when they saw a patient with a broken leg dressed as a knight? "Don't worry, we'll fix your armor in no time!"

11. What did the doctor say to the patient who had a fear of palindromes? "You're fine, it's just a racecar."

12. Why did the doctor become a stand-up comedian? They wanted to make their patients laugh while they got better.

13. Why did the doctor become a math teacher? They wanted to keep things in proportion.

14. What do you call a doctor who only works on the left side of the body? A southpaw-ologist.

15. Why did the doctor join a band? They wanted to give a medical degree of funk.

16. What did the doctor say when the patient asked for their astrological sign? "I'm sorry, I'm an MD, not a mystic."

17. Why did the doctor switch to gardening? They wanted to keep their patients healthy from the root up.

18. Why did the doctor give up on baking? Their patients kept getting muffin-top disease.

19. Why did the doctor become a taxi driver? They wanted to offer bedside transport.

20. What did the doctor say to the patient with a broken nose? "Well, it looks like you're smelling what I'm stepping in."

21. Why did the doctor become a photographer? They wanted to develop their skills.

22. Why did the doctor become an athlete? They wanted to work on their physical therapy skills.

23. Why did the doctor switch to painting? They wanted to cure the blues.

24. Why did the doctor join a band? They wanted to cure the blues.

25. Why did the doctor become a magician? They wanted to have a few tricks up their sleeve.

26. Why did the doctor become a pilot? They wanted to take off in their career.

27. Why did the doctor become a film director? They wanted to call the shots.

28. Why did the doctor become a gardener? They wanted to see things grow and flourish.

29. Why did the doctor become a chef? They wanted to whip up some tasty cures.

30. What did the doctor say to the patient with a broken foot? "Looks like you're out for a walk."

31. Why did the doctor become a hairdresser? They wanted to give their patients a new look.

32. Why did the doctor become a scientist? They wanted to experiment with new cures.

33. Why did the doctor become a fashion designer? They wanted to make their patients look good and feel better.

34. Why did the doctor become a detective? They wanted to investigate their patients

35. Why did the doctor become a musician? They wanted to play the right notes to cure their patients.

36. Why did the doctor become a zookeeper? They wanted to study animal cures.

37. Why did the doctor become a mathematician? They wanted to calculate the perfect dose.

38. Why did the doctor become a sailor? They wanted to chart new medical waters.

39. Why did the doctor become a computer programmer? They wanted to debug medical software.

40. What did the doctor say to the patient with a sore throat? "Looks like you're feeling a bit under the weather."

41. Why did the doctor become a therapist? They wanted to heal the mind as well as the body.

42. Why did the doctor become a teacher? They wanted to educate their patients about health.

43. Why did the doctor become a writer? They wanted to pen the perfect prescription.

44. Why did the doctor become a comedian? They wanted to make medicine funny.

45. Why did the doctor become a detective? They wanted to solve medical mysteries.

46. Why did the doctor become a gardener? They wanted to cultivate a healthy lifestyle.

47. Why did the doctor become a chef? They wanted to cook up some tasty cures.

48. Why did the doctor become a musician? They wanted to play the right notes to heal their patients.

49. Why did the doctor become a zookeeper? They wanted to study animal cures.

50. What did the doctor say to the patient with a broken arm? "Looks like you'll have to give me a hand with this one."

51. Why did the doctor become a mechanic? They wanted to fix what was broken.

52. Why did the doctor become a astronaut? They wanted to reach new heights in medicine.

53. Why did the doctor become a firefighter? They wanted to put out medical emergencies.

54. Why did the doctor become a construction worker? They wanted to build a better healthcare system.

55. Why did the doctor become a journalist? They wanted to report on medical breakthroughs.

56. Why did the doctor become a chef? They wanted to serve up some healthy dishes.

57. Why did the doctor become a farmer? They wanted to cultivate a healthy lifestyle.

58. Why did the doctor become a musician? They wanted to play the right notes to cure their patients.

59. Why did the doctor become a zookeeper? They wanted to study animal cures.

60. What did the doctor say to the patient with a broken finger? "Looks like you'll have to give me a hand with this one."

61. Why did the doctor become a lawyer? They wanted to fight for medical rights.

62. Why did the doctor become a personal trainer? They wanted to help their patients get fit.

63. Why did the doctor become a painter? They wanted to create a picture of health.

64. Why did the doctor become a race car driver? They wanted to speed up their medical career.

65. Why did the doctor become a rock climber? They wanted to climb to the top of their medical field.

66. Why did the doctor become a pilot? They wanted to soar to new medical heights.

67. Why did the doctor become a detective? They wanted to solve medical mysteries.

68. Why did the doctor become a gardener? They wanted to cultivate a healthy lifestyle.

69. Why did the doctor become a chef? They wanted to cook up some tasty cures.

70. What did the doctor say to the patient with a stomachache? "Looks like you've got a lot on your plate."

71. Why did the doctor become a mechanic? They wanted to fix what was broken.

72. Why did the doctor become an astronaut? They wanted to reach new heights in medicine.

73. Why did the doctor become a firefighter? They wanted to put out medical emergencies.

74. Why did the doctor become a construction worker? They wanted to build a better healthcare system.

75. Why did the doctor become a journalist? They wanted to report on medical breakthroughs.

76. Why did the doctor become a chef? They wanted to serve up some healthy dishes.

77. Why did the doctor become a farmer? They wanted to cultivate a healthy lifestyle.

78. Why did the doctor become a musician? They wanted to play the right notes to cure their patients.

79. Why did the doctor become a zookeeper? They wanted to study animal cures.

80. What did the doctor say to the patient with a broken leg? "Looks like you're hopping mad."

81. Why did the doctor become a politician? They wanted to make healthcare a top priority.

82. Why did the doctor become a fashion designer? They wanted to dress up medical care.

83. Why did the doctor become a magician? They wanted to make medical problems disappear.

84. Why did the doctor become a librarian? They wanted to prescribe the right books for their patients.

85. Why did the doctor become a race car driver? They wanted to speed up their medical career.

86. Why did the doctor become a pilot? They wanted to soar to new medical heights.

87. Why did the doctor become a detective? They wanted to solve medical mysteries.

88. Why did the doctor become a gardener? They wanted to cultivate a healthy lifestyle.

89. Why did the doctor become a chef? They wanted to cook up some tasty cures.

90. What did the doctor say to the patient with a headache? "Looks like you're feeling a little brain-dead."

91. Why did the doctor become a painter? They wanted to create a picture of health.

92. Why did the doctor become a personal trainer? They wanted to help their patients get fit.

93. Why did the doctor become a comedian? They wanted to make medicine funny.

94. Why did the doctor become a musician? They wanted to play the right notes to cure their patients.

95. Why did the doctor become a zookeeper? They wanted to study animal cures.

96. Why did the doctor become a writer? They wanted to pen the perfect prescription.

97. Why did the doctor become a detective? They wanted to solve medical mysteries.

98. Why did the doctor become a gardener? They wanted to cultivate a healthy lifestyle.

99. Why did the doctor become a chef? They wanted to cook up some tasty cures.

100. What did the doctor say to the patient who was a hypochondriac? "You're making me sick!"

101. Why did the doctor go on vacation? They needed a little "me-time."

102. Why did the doctor get into the medical field? They wanted to help others.

103. What did the doctor say when they found out they had a patient who was a comedian? "Looks like I'll be the one prescribing the laughs this time."

104. What do you call a doctor who fixes websites? A URLologist.

105. Why did the doctor become an actor? They wanted to play a leading role in healthcare.

106. Why did the doctor become a singer? They wanted to sing the praises of modern medicine.

107. Why did the doctor become a tailor? They wanted to stitch up their patients' wounds.

108. What do you call a doctor who always has a backup plan? A stethoscope-er.

109. Why did the doctor become a fisherman? They wanted to catch some healthy fish for their patients.

110. What did the doctor say when their patient asked them to heal their broken heart? "I'm a doctor, not a magician!"

111. Why did the doctor become a personal shopper? They wanted to help their patients find the perfect healthcare products.

112. Why did the doctor become a basketball player? They wanted to give their patients a shot at health.

113. What do you call a doctor who only sees patients at night? A nocturnal practitioner.

114. Why did the doctor become a chef? They wanted to cook up some healthy dishes for their patients.

115. What do you call a doctor who specializes in treating sick computers? A virusologist.

116. Why did the doctor become a farmer? They wanted to grow some healthy crops for their patients.

117. What do you call a doctor who always seems to be on the phone? A cell-ular practitioner.

118. Why did the doctor become a designer? They wanted to create the perfect medical devices.

119. Why did the doctor become a hairstylist? They wanted to give their patients a cut above the rest.

120. What did the doctor say when their patient asked for a second opinion? "Okay, let me check with my multiple personalities first."

121. Why did the doctor become a skydiver? They wanted to take a leap of faith in their medical career.

122. Why did the doctor become a police officer? They wanted to put the cuffs on sickness.

123. What do you call a doctor who never says no? A yes-ician.

124. Why did the doctor become a rock climber? They wanted to scale new medical heights.

125. Why did the doctor become a chef? They wanted to cook up some healthy food for their patients.

126. What do you call a doctor who always takes the scenic route? A scenic practitioner.

127. Why did the doctor become a translator? They wanted to speak the language of medicine.

128. Why did the doctor become a tailor? They wanted to sew up their patients' health problems.

129. Why did the doctor become a mechanic? They wanted to fix any medical problems that arose.

130. What did the doctor say when their patient asked them for a miracle? "Sorry, I'm a doctor, not a miracle worker."

131. Why did the doctor become a firefighter? They wanted to put out medical emergencies.

132. Why did the doctor become a construction worker? They wanted to build a better healthcare system.

133. Why did the doctor become a journalist? They wanted to report on medical breakthroughs.

134. Why did the doctor become a zookeeper? They wanted to study animal cures.

135. Why did the doctor become a musician? They wanted to play the right notes to cure their patients.

136. Why did the doctor become a detective? They wanted to solve medical mysteries.

137. Why did the doctor become a lifeguard? They wanted to save lives on and off the beach.

138. Why did the doctor become a personal trainer? They wanted to whip their patients into healthy shape.

139. What do you call a doctor who always carries a pen and paper? A scriptologist.

140. Why did the doctor become a racecar driver? They wanted to speed up their patients' recovery time.

141. What do you call a doctor who always makes their patients laugh? A giggle practitioner.

142. Why did the doctor become a gardener? They wanted to plant the seeds of health in their patients.

143. Why did the doctor become a therapist? They wanted to heal their patients' minds as well as their bodies.

144. Why did the doctor become a librarian? They wanted to prescribe the perfect medical literature.

145. What do you call a doctor who always wears sunglasses? A sun-ologist.

146. Why did the doctor become a pilot? They wanted to soar to new medical heights.

147. Why did the doctor become a magician? They wanted to make their patients' ailments disappear.

148. What do you call a doctor who always has a joke up their sleeve? A humor-ologist.

149. Why did the doctor become a teacher? They wanted to educate their patients on health and wellness.

150. Why did the doctor become a postal worker? They wanted to deliver healthy care packages to their patients.

151. Why did the doctor become a magician? They wanted to make their patients' ailments disappear.

152. What do you call a doctor who always has a joke up their sleeve? A humor-ologist.

153. Why did the doctor become a teacher? They wanted to educate their patients on health and wellness.

154. Why did the doctor become a postal worker? They wanted to deliver healthy care packages to their patients.

155. Why did the doctor become a professional athlete? They wanted to showcase the benefits of staying healthy.

156. What do you call a doctor who always takes a break? A rest-ician.

157. Why did the doctor become a geologist? They wanted to study the minerals and vitamins in rocks.

158. Why did the doctor become a motivational speaker? They wanted to inspire their patients to live healthier lives.

159. What do you call a doctor who specializes in treating pets? A vet-ician.

160. Why did the doctor become a plumber? They wanted to unclog any medical issues.

161. Why did the doctor become a teacher? They wanted to teach their patients about the importance of staying healthy.

162. Why did the doctor become a writer? They wanted to write the book on medical success.

163. Why did the doctor become a gardener? They wanted to cultivate health in their patients.

164. What do you call a doctor who always has a funny story to share? A humor-ician.

165. Why did the doctor become a librarian? They wanted to read up on the latest medical research.

166. Why did the doctor become a masseuse? They wanted to rub out any health problems.

167. Why did the doctor become a weatherman? They wanted to predict and prevent medical issues.

168. What do you call a doctor who always brings a smile to their patients' faces? A smile-ician.

169. Why did the doctor become a lawyer? They wanted to defend their patients' right to health.

170. Why did the doctor become a painter? They wanted to paint a healthy picture for their patients.

171. Why did the doctor become a plumber? They wanted to unclog any medical issues.

172. What do you call a doctor who always has a positive outlook? A hope-ician.

173. Why did the doctor become a travel agent? They wanted to help their patients plan healthy vacations.

174. Why did the doctor become a musician? They wanted to play a healthy tune.

175. What do you call a doctor who always has a friendly ear to listen? A hear-ician.

176. Why did the doctor become a chef? They wanted to cook up healthy recipes for their patients.

177. Why did the doctor become a firefighter? They wanted to put out any medical emergencies.

178. What do you call a doctor who always has a positive attitude? A positivity-ician.

179. Why did the doctor become a personal shopper? They wanted to help their patients pick out healthy food choices.

180. Why did the doctor become a florist? They wanted to give their patients a healthy dose of nature.

181. Why did the doctor become a firefighter? They wanted to put out any medical emergencies.

182. What do you call a doctor who always has a healthy tip? A wellness-ician.

183. Why did the doctor become a movie star? They wanted to show how health can make you shine.

184. Why did the doctor become a scientist? They wanted to discover new medical breakthroughs.

185. What do you call a doctor who always has a kind word? A kind-ician.

186. Why did the doctor become a park ranger? They wanted to promote healthy outdoor activities for their patients.

187. Why did the doctor become a fashion designer? They wanted to create healthy and stylish clothing for their patients.

188. What do you call a doctor who always has a solution? A solve-ician.

189. Why did the doctor become a beach volleyball player? They wanted to promote healthy exercise in the sun.

190. Why did the doctor become a fisherman? They wanted to catch the healthiest fish for their patients.

191. Why did the doctor become a fashion designer? They wanted to create healthy and stylish clothing for their patients.

192. What do you call a doctor who always has a bright idea? A brilliance-ician.

193. Why did the doctor become a pilot? They wanted to fly to the healthiest destinations.

194. Why did the doctor become a detective? They wanted to uncover any medical mysteries.

195. What do you call a doctor who always has a listening ear? A listen-ician.

196. Why did the doctor become a zookeeper? They wanted to observe and learn from healthy animals.

197. Why did the doctor become a chef? They wanted to create healthy and delicious meals for their patients.

198. What do you call a doctor who always has a plan? A strateg-ician.

199. Why did the doctor become a farmer? They wanted to grow healthy fruits and vegetables for their patients.

200.   Why did the doctor become a comedian? They wanted to make their patients laugh their way to good health.